Loraine Araújo
Lorena Araújo

Burnout Syndrome and its Implications for Nursing

Loraine Araújo
Lorena Araújo

Burnout Syndrome and its Implications for Nursing

The challenge in the contemporary world

ScienciaScripts

Imprint

Any brand names and product names mentioned in this book are subject to trademark, brand or patent protection and are trademarks or registered trademarks of their respective holders. The use of brand names, product names, common names, trade names, product descriptions etc. even without a particular marking in this work is in no way to be construed to mean that such names may be regarded as unrestricted in respect of trademark and brand protection legislation and could thus be used by anyone.

Cover image: www.ingimage.com

This book is a translation from the original published under ISBN 978-620-2-19041-1.

Publisher:
Sciencia Scripts
is a trademark of
Dodo Books Indian Ocean Ltd. and OmniScriptum S.R.L publishing group

120 High Road, East Finchley, London, N2 9ED, United Kingdom
Str. Armeneasca 28/1, office 1, Chisinau MD-2012, Republic of Moldova, Europe
Printed at: see last page
ISBN: 978-620-7-15799-0

INDICE

1 INTRODUCTION

In contemporary life, work plays an essential role in surviving and maintaining economic standards that allow for well-being in society. It determines social *status*, bringing prestige and respect within the cultural standards to which it belongs. It also provides meaning to life, satisfying psychosocial needs and significantly influencing the physical and mental health of individuals (MOURAO et al, 2017).

However, the transformations that the globalized world has undergone have significantly changed the working environment, where competitiveness and productivity have become a market necessity. The relentless pursuit of different activities has led to an increase in workloads, leading to the appearance of physical, psychological and emotional ailments.

Nowadays, there is a growing emphasis on economic value to the detriment of human capital, and it is possible to see the consequences in daily work life through the reduced autonomy of workers, unequal pay among professional staff, work overload, lack of recognition and teamwork and the existence of a conflict of values between the organization and the worker (FRANCA, F et al, 2012).

These changes in the world of work, resulting from the incorporation of new technologies, have given workers new skills and abilities, both in the ways of managing, organizing, planning and using services, and in the relationships established between workers, managers and the people who use the services (FRANCA, S et al, 2012).

The skills expected of workers are those in which they are able to act in situations of constant transformation at work, identify problems, propose solutions, self-educate, be creative and work as part of a team, with a view to optimizing productivity. All of this has required efforts that have worn workers down physically and psychologically, generating stress, since they are not prepared for such changes (BARRETO et al, 2012). In this scenario, workers are required to produce and qualify, which can lead to wear and tear and stress, seriously impacting workers' health, substantially reducing their quality of life and affecting the provision of health services (MOURAO et al., 2017).

Thus, work does not always bring fulfillment and professional satisfaction, and the organization and working conditions are determining factors for the emergence of work-related illnesses, including Burnout Syndrome (LIMA; FARAH;

BUSTAMANTE-TEIXEIRA, 2018).

Burnout syndrome is a special type of chronic and prolonged occupational stress resulting from an imbalance between demand and the individual's ability to respond, mainly due to interpersonal demands at work. It is evidenced by a progressive loss of energy, idealism and expectations that occurs in workers who generally work in professional areas of help, being a general malaise that leads to damage to their productivity and satisfaction in relation to their work (GREGORY; MENSER, 2015).

Health professionals seem to be one of the most susceptible to the syndrome because of their exposure to the risks and burdens inherent in the profession. And among health professionals, nursing is the profession that experiences the most stress and the syndrome.

Nursing, as a social practice, has not been exempt from the novelties arising from this process of globalization, such as long working hours, insufficient numbers of staff, lack of professional recognition, high exposure to biological and physical risks, as well as constant contact with suffering, pain and often death.

These workers have the job of constantly caring for patients and, in this context, often witness cases of death and bereavement, being exposed to the emotional tensions of such events (MEDEIROS-COSTA et al., 2017). As a consequence of these stressors, the professional is led to a lack of motivation, alienation, depression, fatigue, frustration, suffering, impotence, stress and Burnout (BEZERRA; BERESIN, 2009).

According to Decree No. 3.048 of May 6, 1999, which deals with pathogenic agents that cause occupational or work-related illnesses, Burnout syndrome is included in the list of occupational and work-related illnesses (Ministerio da Saude, Portaria No. 1339/1999).

It is classified under Work-Related Mental and Behavioural Disorders under code Z73.0 (Group V of the International Classification of Diseases, 10th revision - ICD-10), recognized as an occupational risk for professions involving health care, education and human services (MINISTERIO DA SAUDE, 2001).

Burnout, also known as professional burnout, can be considered a major problem in today's professional world, where economic values are increasingly prioritized to the detriment of human values. It has been affecting workers since the end of the last century and continues into this new millennium, implying transformations in social and working relationships (ARAUJO et al., 2007).

Burnout indicates "lack of energy", signaling the limit of the worker's physical and mental capacity for work, due to the excessive effort employed in work activities. Burnout syndrome occurs as a reaction to work-related stress in which the worker loses the sense of their relationship with work and becomes disinterested in their usual activities (LIMA; FARAH; BUSTAMANTE-TEIXEIRA, 2018).

Although Burnout is recognized as an occupational risk for nursing, it is still a disease of which the general population and the affected professionals have little knowledge. This lack of information leads to the worsening of symptoms, increasing the number of absences from work, as well as contributing to the underreporting of the disease (MEDEIROS-COSTA et al, 2017).

Considering the importance of this issue in the current capitalist scenario, together with the reduced scientific production and information in the field of workers' health. The purpose of this review is to present some aspects of Burnout syndrome and its relationship with nursing work, highlighting its causes and consequences for the social and professional health of workers.

2 THEORETICAL BACKGROUND

Conceptual Aspects

Conceptually, the term Burnout, derived from the English language, is defined as something that, due to a lack of energy and exhaustion, has ceased to function. Burnout syndrome, identified in the 1970s, was first described by Freudenberger and Maslach in the 1920s, providing the first description of the phenomenon. It is also known as professional burnout and can be interpreted as "burning out" (TRIGO; TENG; HALLAK, 2007).

Burn means to burn out, *out* means outside, exhaustion. *Burnout* indicates that the professional's exhaustion has already exceeded the permissible limits. Generally speaking, it means something that has completely burned out, ceasing to function due to an absolute lack of energy.

Burnout is a defense response, however inappropriate, to the chronification of emotional and interpersonal stress at work that has reached intolerable limits (FERNANDES et al., 2017). It signals the limit of the physical and mental capacity available for the activity, to the extent that the energy invested has been swollen, without the expected financial or personal return. It is characterized as a psychosocial phenomenon, the result of the inability to adapt as a response to coping with stressors.

Burnout, therefore, stems from an imbalance in which the levels of demands and expectations exceed resources and reality and prevent the individual from adapting to the situation experienced. As a result, workers develop a gradual loss of energy, commitment and hope, causing damage to productivity and job satisfaction (LIMA; FARAH; BUSTAMANTE-TEIXEIRA, 2018).

Burnout syndrome is insidious and occurs mainly in individuals committed to their profession, who work in conditions of psychological demand associated with low decision-making power (TRIGO; TENG; HALLAK, 2007). Although Burnout Syndrome is seen in all professions, it affects workers whose work is considered to be caring and involves interpersonal contact. Professionals in the fields of education, health, social assistance, human resources, prison guards, firefighters, police officers and women who work double shifts are at greater risk of developing the disorder, and it is particularly evident in those whose work involves high levels of stress, especially in the health sector, including nursing, regardless of their occupation.

Nurses, technicians and nursing assistants working in direct patient care sectors had a higher prevalence of unsatisfactory quality of life at work than those working in exclusively administrative sectors or in support and indirect care services.

This difference in prevalence is statistically significant specifically for professionals working in inpatient units for highly dependent or critically ill patients, such as the Surgical Center, the Medical and Neurological Clinics and the Intensive Care Unit.

Working in these sectors is often linked to situations such as a fast pace of work, a greater demand for physical effort in patient care and the need for speed and agility in decision-making.

Thus, working in these sectors can be a stressful situation for nursing workers, contributing to the occurrence of problems such as occupational stress and musculoskeletal disorders, which can have a negative impact on the physiological, psychological, relational and organizational spheres that make up quality of life at work (AZEVEDO; NERY; CARDOSO, 2017). According to Bucasio et al. (2006), Burnout Syndrome affects 10% of nursing workers in Brazil, making it a social problem. This is due to the inherent characteristics of the profession, such as living with others, intense emotional interaction and unavailability for leisure activities and holidays, as well as the transformations in the world of work (RITTER; STUMM; KIRCHER, 2009).

These professionals who work in helping roles, unlike others, are more susceptible to developing Burnout Syndrome because they are faced with three levels: the ills of society, the needs of the individuals who seek out these professionals and the needs of themselves, producing negative consequences from an individual, professional, family and social perspective (MOURAO et al., 2017).

In addition, factors such as high service demands, work overload, double shifts, occupational hazards, precarious material resources, lack of qualified staff and conflicting interpersonal relationships make this category more vulnerable. Progressive exposure to these stressors leads to physical and emotional exhaustion, interfering with quality of life and impairing interaction with their functions and the work environment that trigger this syndrome (FERNANDES et al., 2017).

In addition to work overload, the monthly salary can be a significant factor in professionals' need to supplement their income by working in other institutions, which is quite common among health workers. This requires the professional to work in various roles every week, sometimes different ones, subjecting them to the demands and pressures of various workplaces (LUZ et al., 2017).

All these factors can contribute to the development of feelings of demotivation, dissatisfaction and disillusionment in the professional in relation to their work, since the working conditions offered affect the quality of life of the worker and the quality of the service offered to users.

Burnout syndrome is characterized by three main symptom dimensions, which are independent but can be associated: emotional exhaustion, depersonalization and personal dissatisfaction.

The first is verified by a lack of energy and enthusiasm, fatigue and emotional and/or physical exhaustion. It presents itself as a direct manifestation of individual stress, with externalized feelings of being stretched beyond one's limits, with a deterioration in the individual's physical and emotional resources to deal with the stressful situation, to which can be added feelings of frustration and tension. It is sometimes seen as the most important and central factor in the syndrome.

<u>Depersonalization</u> or cynicism, observed through emotional insensitivity, is linked to the interpersonal conjuncture of the syndrome, in which negative attitudes are directed towards the people who receive the work. Depersonalization is characterized as a loss of compassion and unconcern for other people, leading the professional to treat patients, colleagues and the organization in a dehumanized way (FERNANDES et al., 2017).

Lastly, <u>low personal satisfaction</u> or feelings of incompetence are related to the individual's negative assessments of their performance at work and their future in that profession (BEZERRA et al, 2017).

It refers to the perception of a deterioration in one's ability and dissatisfaction with one's achievements and successes at work, making one unhappy with one's professional development, with a consequent decline in one's sense of competence and success, as well as in one's ability to interact socially.

According to Jodas and Haddad (2009, p. 193)

Burnout syndrome is the emotional response to chronic stress as a result of intense work relationships with other people, or of professionals who have high expectations of their professional development and dedication to their profession and fail to achieve the expected return.

Burnout causes negative attitudes and feelings in relation to the activities carried out at work, such as dissatisfaction, frustration, demotivation, emotional exhaustion, inefficiency and dehumanization or cynicism (ABRANCHES; MUROFUSE; NAPOLEAO, 2005).

In other words, for workers with burnout, the meaning of their relationship with work is lost; work activities cease to be important; and any effort at work seems pointless, indicating a breakdown, which comes after all the available energy has been used up.

In this perspective, the problem of burnout related to turnover, i.e. the turnover of professionals in the organization, in nursing, due to leaving or abandoning the profession, for example, is a worldwide concern, both in Western and Eastern countries, especially in the USA and China. Studies show a concern with this issue in various areas of nursing, such as clinical medicine, intensive care, management and administration of nursing services (SILVA; NORA; OLIVEIRA, 2017).

The syndrome is recognized as an occupational psychopathology (Group V of ICD-10) and is included in Annex II of Article 2 of Decree 6.957/1999, governed by the Social Security system.

Incidence of Burnout Syndrome

In Brazil, little research has been carried out on the subject, but the data is worrying: an investigation carried out by the *International Stress Management Association* (ISMA-BR, 2006), points out that 70% of Brazilians suffer the consequences of stress, of which 30% are victims of *Burnout.*

Despite underreporting, Burnout Syndrome affects many workers. According to the

Ministry of Social Security, it is estimated that 4.2 million people were taken off work in 2007, of which 3,852 were diagnosed with *Burnout* Syndrome (GONCALVES, 2008).

According to studies, this syndrome generally affects individuals who have never previously presented any psychopathological alteration and they establish a relationship between the incidence of Burnout and length of service, age, gender, marital status, presence of children and area of work.

In relation to length of service, studies have shown that people with a higher level of education are more prone to burnout, affecting mainly professionals at the beginning of their career, with it being more common with up to three years of professional activity (HADDAD; JODAS, 2009).

The high level of education of individuals can be a contributor to stress due to the high expectation of performance that hovers around these professionals, leading to greater demands for responsibility in team leadership, which denotes a concern on the part of professionals to acquire greater knowledge and security to support their actions (LUZ et al., 2017).

With regard to the length of time they have been working in the profession, this can be explained by the fact that, at the moment, these younger professionals, with little experience and recent training, are in a phase of transition between perspective and reality, in which idealized expectations are not always realized in the reality of daily practice.

In addition, young people are more idealistic and prone to disillusionment, they feel unprepared to take on the responsibilities of the profession and may suffer from an identity crisis due to a lack of socialization at work (LIMA; FARAH; BUSTAMANTE-TEIXEIRA, 2018).

For researchers, because they are recent graduates who don't have the confidence and professional qualifications that the area requires, it makes the individual unstable in their work, causing fear, thus contributing to the stressor for *Burnout* Syndrome (SIMOES; BIANCHI, 2016).

On the other hand, professionals with longer careers are considered to be more experienced and mature in terms of coping with stressors, and are more adapted to them, which possibly makes them more self-confident and skillful in their practice and less prone to Burnout Syndrome. With regard to age, it is believed that the fact that individuals over the age of thirty are protected from Burnout Syndrome may be related to the so-called 'healthy worker effect', a phenomenon that occurs due to individuals giving up and fleeing their profession, with only healthy employees remaining (LIMA; FARAH; BUSTAMANTE-TEIXEIRA, 2018).

However, research has also shown that long years of being subjected to the demands of the job could lead to the onset of the syndrome as a result of chronic wear and tear due to the length of service. The longer the length of service in a given area, the greater the level of stress, and there is therefore a significantly high correlation between stress and length of service in the area (LUZ et al., 2017).

In relation to gender, research shows that there is a higher prevalence of emotional exhaustion in women, which is possibly related to the fact that most of them are nursing staff, a professional category historically performed by women. It is also due to the double workload (domestic and professional activities), usually performed by women, which overloads them physically.

While men are more related to depersonalization, since they have more instrumental attitudes and are less emotionally responsive (TAMAYO, 2009).

Another point to highlight is the fact that single people without children are more likely to suffer from the disease. According to Haddad and Jodas (2009), this is possibly because married professionals are more mature and stable. In other words, with family life, the individual develops better interpersonal relationships.

Singles, on the other hand, may feel the emptiness of the absence of emotional lakes and the need for a family relationship that brings stability and companionship (LUZ et al., 2017).

It should be emphasized here that it is not enough to have a stable emotional relationship, but the quality of this relationship must be taken into account, otherwise it can act inversely as a stressor (LUZ et al., 2017).

The association of motherhood/paternity is related to greater responsibility, maturity and more realistic expectations. It can be deduced that the possible stability generated by the emotional satisfaction of being a parent or responsible for a family may be possible external factors for lower stress levels in married people.

In relation to the area of work, nursing professionals in clinical areas experience Burnout Syndrome more frequently than their supervisors, which indicates that care areas provide a greater stress load and, consequently, increase the incidence of the syndrome (SILVA; NORA; OLIVEIRA, 2017).

Burnout and Depression

Burnout syndrome and depression have several "qualitative" characteristics in common, especially in the more severe forms of Burnout, according to Lacovides (2003). However, some differences can be established between them. Bucasio et al. reaffirm Freudenberger's idea that the "depressive state" present in Burnout is temporary and oriented towards a specific situation in the person's life (in this case, work).

Furthermore, Maslach, Schaufeli and Leiter, in 2001, reported that Burnout only affects the professional field, while depression affects all areas of the individual's life. Another difference would be that in Burnout, the feeling of guilt, characteristic of depression, would not be present and the symptoms of indecisiveness and inactivity would be related to fatigue, unlike depression, which would be related to the illness itself (BUCASIO et al., 2006).

The nature of the Burnout/depression association is not yet well known, but it is known that it may be due to common etiological antecedents, and that Burnout may be a phase (or a precursor) in the development of a depressive disorder (BUCASIO et al., 2006).

Often, people with the syndrome are diagnosed with depression or another mental disorder, without the proper link to work, contributing to a delay in the correct treatment for these professionals or often underreporting of the illness (MEDEIROS-COSTA et al, 2017).

Risk Factors

The current market situation, characterized by high organizational competitiveness, makes human work one of the main differentiators for the quality of services. As a result, new work routines, skills and involvement needs are being demanded of workers, often pushing them to the limits of emotional and professional exhaustion.

This shows how important it is to understand aspects related to human behavior in the context of workers' health, such as diagnosing stressors that can compromise results and individual health (SCHUSTER; DIAS, 2018).

Hospital organizations have been characterized by the need for individual and complex responses, requiring new skills from professionals, who are faced with technological changes and the demands of their clientele, often causing transformations in their work process.

The literature frequently mentions the pressure of performing activities and the extreme stress of professionals as a result of carrying out daily activities. The stressful characteristics of such activities are attributed, among other things, to the reduction in the number of professionals working in nursing and the increase in voluntary job abandonment rates (SILVA; NORA; OLIVEIRA, 2017).

The strong demand for excellent results and the close monitoring of workers' performance, even when the tasks are carried out to their satisfaction, without taking into account the real difficulties faced by the professional in carrying out their work, creates an environment full of paradoxical injunctions, of demands that are mutually exclusive.

While everyone is required to achieve excellence, the increasingly demanding evaluation processes mean that even workers who meet all the productivity criteria are only average (LUZ et al., 2017). Working conditions pose risks to people's safety, since the lack of equipment needed for care means that their safety targets are not being followed correctly.

This exposes professionals to various risks, both for themselves and for patients, leading to health problems or accidents at work, as well as a sense of incompleteness (WORM et al, 2016).

A work environment that lacks resources, appreciation and satisfaction, for example, is a risk factor for Burnout Syndrome.

Factors such as fatigue, physical and mental exhaustion, combined with job dissatisfaction and suffering, generate emotional exhaustion for the nursing team in order to cope with their own suffering and the demands of the hospital organization. This emotional work, which is the conscious and unconscious effort of the worker to adapt to the demands of the organization and the work environment, appeared to be an important factor in causing burnout and turnover (SILVA; NORA; OLIVEIRA, 2017).

This is especially the case in sectors such as intensive care units, which require a high emotional workload because they deal with critical patient care situations and technical demands, showing a significant relationship with burnout and turnover.

Workers' perception of the discrepancy between their efforts and the objectives achieved at work can generate a series of feelings of frustration and interpersonal stress. If exposure to these elements occurs for a prolonged period of time, it can favor the development of Burnout (SCHUSTER; DIAS, 2018).

It is known that this is influenced by external factors related to work, as well as internal or personal factors that contribute and make the individual more vulnerable to triggering the syndrome. Among the internal factors are personality, individual temperament and the individual's ability to manage the stress and emotional demands of patients and their families (BUCASIO et al., 2006).

According to Benevides-Pereira (2002), personal characteristics play the role of facilitators or inhibitors of the action of stressors. People who are more competitive, hard-working, impatient, with an excessive need for control, difficulty tolerating frustration and low self-esteem are generally more susceptible to developing Burnout Syndrome. Thus, people who are very involved with their work and who have these personality traits are at greater risk of developing the syndrome.

Because it depends on individual characteristics, it is a reality made up of subjective experiences that usually involve negative behavior in the face of stressful situations.

Research shows that work organization has a strong influence on the psychic apparatus of workers and that, after conflicting experiences, the subject may gradually wear out, resulting in a symptomatology that substantially degrades the professional's quality of life

(MOURAO et al., 2017).

External factors are those directly linked to the organizational structure of nursing work and professional practice, and according to some studies are more closely related to Burnout Syndrome (TAMAYO, 2009).

These stressors are linked to the physical environment, the demands of the work itself, the performance of the job and the components of the organizational structure of the work environment (JESUS et al., 2017).

These include the accumulation of nurses' responsibilities in their day-to-day work; the excessive workload; night shifts and long working hours at an intense pace; overtime; pressure to make quick decisions and little rest, coupled with the reduced number of professionals and material resources.

Other studies also point to frequent interruptions during the execution of their tasks, the simultaneity of performing different tasks, not having enough time to give emotional support to the patient or the lack of time for some patients who need care as important stressors (JESUS et al., 2017).

According to Ritter, Stumm and Kircher (2009), these factors cause alterations to their sleep, eating and social activity biorhythms, restricting social and family life, predisposing workers to different occupational stressors that directly affect their well-being.

The work environment puts the worker in stressful situations, with exposure to biological risks; psychic overload due to dealing with patients who are usually seriously ill; as well as continuous and direct contact with the suffering, pain and death of patients, which often requires greater emotional control than in other professions, making these professionals more prone to developing Burnout Syndrome (RITTER; STUMM; KIRCHER, 2009).

In addition, these professionals are still closer, most of the time at work, to patients, their families and their realities, feeling charged and pressured to respond to their needs (LIMA; FARAH; BUSTAMANTE- TEIXEIRA, 2018).

In this way, it can be seen that, regardless of the specialties in which they work, these professionals deal directly with biopsychosocial phenomena related to the process of patients becoming ill, involving, in this interpersonal relationship, situations of stress, anxiety, fear and emotional tension, such as pain, fragility, suffering and, in many cases, death (MOURAO, 2017).

It is worth noting that the increased responsibility in the workplace, the disproportionality between the number of patients and nursing staff, as well as multiple jobs can generate more workloads and greater tension among workers (AZEVEDO; NERY; CARDOSO, 2017).

These factors subject nursing workers to multiple demands which, in addition to unfavorable working conditions, have an impact on their health.

Difficulties in delimiting the different roles between nurses, technicians and nursing assistants, as well as competitiveness between professionals, generate conflicts and difficulties in interpersonal relationships in the workplace. The lack of autonomy and relationships between the medical and nursing staff, as well as the lack of organizational support from management and their negative assessment of the professionals, creates an environment that can potentially generate conflicts (PADILLHA et al., 2017).

Among the organizational obstacles that can damage social relations in the workplace, we highlight the impoverishment and repetitiveness of tasks, the lack of motivation and stimulation, the precarious integration between employees and the organization and the psychological impacts of poor management that does not pursue a preventive and humanistic policy.

The literature has shown that support from managers seems to be more important to nursing workers than support from colleagues, although the latter is also associated with job satisfaction.

Nursing requires teamwork to provide quality care, and since social support is a coping strategy often used by these workers, healthy working relationships are important. In addition to support from colleagues and managers, recognition of the work by the organization is also important (AZEVEDO; NERY; CARDOSO, 2017).

The perception of social support at work, a dimension that was later included in the demand-control model to assess social integration, trust in the group and help in carrying out tasks from colleagues and superiors, could act as a protective factor against the negative effects of high-demand jobs, a hypothesis that already has good evidence in the scientific literature.

Other studies have also observed the relationship between social support and satisfaction, motivation, commitment to work and/or intention to leave the organization/profession (AZEVEDO; NERY; CARDOSO, 2017).

The current political situation in which nursing workers find themselves; the lack of recognition, autonomy and appreciation of the profession; the narrowing of the job market; employment instability and unemployment are aggravating factors for nursing professionals, which trigger a feeling of injustice and fear about staying in a job, causing workers to accept these conditions (TAMAYO, 2009).

The correlation between the overwork of nursing professionals means that professional burnout often intensifies as a result of the dedication of these workers, with a lower than expected personal income (WORM et al., 2016). As a result, professionals are forced to have several jobs, causing an additional work overload. Nursing workers are therefore at constant risk of experiencing Burnout Syndrome (BUCASIO et al., 2006).

These stressors, depending on their intensity and duration, together with the lack of social support at work, contribute to making nursing the fourth most stressful profession in the public sector, according to the Health Education Authority (ORTIZ; PLATINO, 1991 Apud ABRANCHES; MUROFUSE; NAPOLEAO, 2005). This reality, coupled with job dissatisfaction, affects the emergence or worsening of burnout, and is a predictor of increased turnover rates, i.e. staying in or leaving a job voluntarily.

There is already robust evidence of an inversely proportional relationship between occupational stress in nursing workers and their perceived job satisfaction.

However, quality of life at work is a broader construct than job satisfaction, it also involves other factors, such as a sense of pride in the work done, job security, recognition for the results achieved, perceived salary, human relationships within the group and the organization, working environment, freedom of decision, among others.

The literature has also pointed out important attitudes and behaviors for work that can be affected by quality of life at work, such as vigor, dedication, motivation, engagement, adaptability to changes in the work environment, creativity, willingness to innovate, and even influence the intention to stay or leave the organization/profession (AZEVEDO; NERY; CARDOSO, 2017).

Research indicates that among the factors related to job dissatisfaction are high workloads, role conflicts and irrational beliefs about oneself. Other causes include incivility, aspects related to the workplace, stress and physical and mental exhaustion.

The quality of patient care appears to be strongly influenced by and positively related to Burnout, and as the number of patients seen increases, so do Burnout rates.

There is also a strong relationship between emotional exhaustion and psychosomatic complaints and work impairment, which are associated with turnover intentions. Furthermore, job satisfaction and its derivative factors such as workload, emotional labor and work climate affect professionals of all ages, from recent graduates to those with more than ten years in the profession.

The shortage of professionals working in nursing is highlighted in research as a global phenomenon and is related to turnover and its determinants, having been reported by the authors of articles from various countries, both Western and Eastern.

Among the factors for the decrease in the search for a nursing career or abandonment of work are the high degree of stress resulting from daily care, salary issues, low personal fulfillment, lack of autonomy, interpersonal difficulties with nursing and medical staff and the high workload, which culminates in dissatisfaction with the career, either during graduation or after graduation (SILVA; NORA; OLIVEIRA, 2017).

Symptoms

The symptoms of Burnout Syndrome can be divided into various physical, psychological, behavioral and defensive disorders, which can be isolated or associated. With regard to Burnout, it must be stressed that it is a disease with serious psychological and physical consequences that affects the individual as a whole and society as a whole.

It is worth noting that the symptoms appear differently in each worker, depending, as already explained, on personality, the way the individual faces and responds to stressful situations and the work environment itself (MOURAO et al., 2017).

Physical symptoms: Fatigue, gradual decrease in energy, difficulty relaxing, exhaustion, loss of motivation, tension and musculoskeletal pain (lumbar or cervical), sleep disorders, headache, gastrointestinal disorders (nausea and vomiting, gastritis and ulcers), neuroendocrine alterations (hyperglycemia, hyperlipidemia), cardiovascular disorders (hypertension and heart attacks), respiratory system disorders (bronchitis, asthma), sexual dysfunctions, skin disorders (itching, herpes, allergies, hair loss), increased susceptibility to diseases due to immunological impairment, among others (HALLAK; TENG; TRIGO, 2007).

- Psychic symptoms: Difficulty concentrating and paying attention, memory alterations, slow thinking, psychic exhaustion, feeling of alienation, impatience, dissatisfaction with work, irritability, discouragement, emotional lability, feeling of powerlessness, difficulty in self-acceptance, low self-esteem, dysphoria, depression, disillusionment, sleep disturbances, distrust, hopelessness, paranoia, worry, anxiety and the feeling that when they have finished their work there are still tasks to be done (HALLAK; TENG; TRIGO, 2007).

Behavioral symptoms: Negligence or excessive scrupulousness; recklessness; irritability; aggressiveness; indifference; difficulty in accepting change and complying with the institution's rules and routines; loss of initiative; depersonalization, in which the individual distances themselves from interpersonal relationships; low professional fulfillment, in which the professional copes with negative feelings about him/herself; propensity to self-risk behaviors such as substance and drug abuse (alcohol, coffee, smoking, tranquilizers, illicit substances); suicidal ideas, among others.

- Defensive Symptoms: Tendency to isolation, distancing from personal relationships, social isolation, loss of interest in work and even leisure, absenteeism, abandonment and frequent job changes and irony (BARBOSA; OLIVEIRA; RIBEIRO, 2010). This behavior works as an escape valve, as the individual blames the feeling of being unwell at work on others. In general, Burnout Syndrome manifests itself slowly, oscillating with varying intensity, in which the individual himself rejects the manifestations perceived by his coworkers.

In the most serious cases, the individual affected by burnout acquires an aversion to their job and starts to avoid it, even not being able to enter or pass through their work area. At this more advanced level of the syndrome, it can be irreversible if the individual doesn't leave work. This stage occurs in between 5 and 10% of Burnout patients (BOFF et al., 2006).

Consequences of Burnout

It is known that Burnout Syndrome causes maladjustments in the individual, social and organizational dimensions, leading the individual to various consequences.

According to Hallak, Teng and Trigo (2007), the individual dimension is related to the signs and symptoms described, reflected in personal suffering.

In the social dimension, it is common for people to distance themselves from family members, children and spouses, causing difficulties in relationships and diminishing responsibilities in the family and social spheres. Tobacco use has been described as a strategy used to reduce or control anxiety levels, in a kind of self-medication. Therefore, in situations of very high stress, which generate anxiety, there is some encouragement to use tobacco as a way of alleviating it (AZEVEDO; NERY; CARDOSO, 2017).

In relation to the organizational dimension, Burnout Syndrome can lead to a reduction in the quality of the service provided and low productivity, as well as poor customer service due to negligence and recklessness, making care prone to errors and subjecting the patient to risks (PORTELA, et al, 2015). There is also the manifestation of emotional insensitivity on the part of the worker, prevailing cynicism and affective dissimulation, implying a situation of abandonment, hopelessness, lack of expectation at work and greater difficulty in coping due to fatigue and the fact that they present a kind of disenchantment. In other words, "the drop in the quality and quantity of work produced is the professional result of burnout" (ABRANCHES; MUROFUSE; NAPOLEAO, p. 256, 2005). And due to a lack of attention and concentration, nursing professionals can also be at risk to themselves, as they are more prone to accidents in the workplace, including biological and physical accidents (HALLAK; TENG; TRIGO, 2007).

The literature shows evidence that high workload, stress, fatigue and professional dissatisfaction are associated with errors. Considering that the environment is complex and stressful, the excessive workload of nurses, the insufficient number of professionals in the team and the high levels of stress and dissatisfaction, as well as the sleep deficit of professionals can be associated with the presence of adverse events and incidents (PADILLHA et al, 2017).

Such disorders can also generate unfavorable responses to the work environment and the institution, such as an increase in the rate of absenteeism and sick leave, generating sick leave and the need for the organization to replace employees, transfers, new hires, new training, among other expenses, causing what is known as turnover (HALLAK; TENG; TRIGO, 2007).

Burnout thus causes time and money losses for the individual, the employer, the economy and the public purse.

Thus, although there have been various social and political advances with regard to protecting workers' lives and health, the preponderance of market and productivist interests stands out, in which the professional is reduced to a work tool and understood as an instrument used under the aegis of the current mode of production (MOURAO et al., 2017).

It is therefore clear that the various public policies need to be implemented more effectively and responsibly by the health authorities and employers. There is an urgent need to adopt preventive measures and control occupational illnesses in order to avoid chaos in the social security sector and in Brazil's economy (MOURAO et al., 2017). It is important to clarify that Burnout Syndrome is not a problem of the individual, but of the social environment in which they perform their activities. Murofuse, Abranches and Napoleao, (2011), point out that Burnout Syndrome is a major current psychosocial problem, arousing the interest and concern of North American and European governmental, business and trade union entities due to the severity of its consequences, both on an individual and organizational level.

The individual's suffering has consequences for both their health and their professional performance, as there are personal and organizational changes and/or dysfunctions, with economic and social repercussions (SIMOES; BIANCHI, 2017). It is necessary to recognize, feel important and value the resources that are fundamental to workers' performance, as these are fundamental human needs for job satisfaction. These factors influence the way individuals see their work (pleasurable or not) and how they deal with their work and their own lives (LIMA; FARAH; BUSTAMANTE-TEIXEIRA, 2018).

In general terms, the term "turnover" refers to the voluntary leaving of a job, and in a broader analysis, its motivation is closely related to Burnout and, in turn, to job dissatisfaction; when job satisfaction increases, Burnout and turnover decrease.

Turnover implies at least three consequences for organizations: potential costs, paralysis of activities in progress, and loss of human resources. International literature highlights that the shortage of nursing professionals and high turnover rates in nursing services are currently a global issue (SILVA; NORA; OLIVEIRA, 2017).

More specifically, international productions show a trend towards a decrease in the number of professionals in various nursing settings, such as care homes for the elderly, medical clinics, psychiatric clinics and intensive care in various parts of the world such as the USA, China, Canada and South Korea.

It should also be noted that nursing is a highly stressful and challenging profession, due to the need for specialization, complexity and demands to deal with emergency situations (SILVA; NORA; OLIVEIRA, 2017).

Research reveals dissatisfaction as a multifactorial problem. People with low levels of satisfaction had a higher prevalence of the syndrome (LIMA; FARAH; BUSTAMANTE-TEIXEIRA, 2018). In practice, this means that the more people who develop Burnout, the greater the risk of an increase in turnover rates. These relationships result in a cycle that undermines the health of professionals, the quality of care and the financial balance of the hospital organization (SILVA; NORA; OLIVEIRA, 2017).

Oldenburg Burnout Inventory: the Burnout Measurement Scale

Due to the effects of Burnout Syndrome on the health of people and organizations, over the years various studies have sought to identify the factors involved in this process of illness.

In 1969, Bradley was the first researcher to introduce the term Burnout to the scientific world, in which he characterized staff burnout as the exhaustion of professionals and proposed organizational alternatives as a solution.

Freudenberger popularized Burnout Syndrome through his 1974 work entitled Staff burnout, in which he studied professionals in a psychiatric clinic who dealt with young drug addicts. At this time, Burnout was widespread, but it was rejected by academic society because it was based on empirical research methods (FALGUERAS et al, 2015).

Subsequently, Christina Maslach and her collaborators introduced Burnout to the academic world and gave credibility to the phenomenon through a series of studies with workers and the creation of the research instrument called the Maslach Burnout Inventory (MBI) MASLACH; SCHAUFELI; LEITER, 2001).

They initially studied health and human services professionals, as they believed that, because they deal with high emotional demands, they might be more prone to burnout. They found three obvious feelings in the subjects' reports: emotional exhaustion, a negative perception of patients and a view of themselves as professionally incompetent (SCHAUFELI; LEITER; MASLACH, 2009).

It was then established that the following dimensions are part of the syndrome: exhaustion, cynicism and professional efficacy. However, other researchers have suggested a two-factor model, which only includes emotional exhaustion and depersonalization.

In the 1980s, this identification of factors led to the development of scales to measure burnout syndrome, including the Burnout Questionnaire for Teachers (CBP) and the Brief Burnout Questionnaire (CBB) by Moreno-Jimenez et. al. (1997); the Copenhagen Burnout Inventory (CBI) by Kristensen et. al. (2005); the Shirom-Melamed Burnout Measure (SMBM) by Shirom and Melamed (2006); the Burnout Measure (BM) by Jones (1980) and the Burnout Characterization Scale by Tamayo and Trocoli (2009).

However, the most widely referenced scales on the subject are the Maslach Burnout Inventory (MBI), developed in the early 1980s by Maslach and Jackson (1981) and the Oldenburg Burnout Inventory (OLBI), created by Evangelia Demerouti in 1999 in Germany and later translated into English.

The MBI is based on a three-dimensional model to measure emotional exhaustion, depersonalization and personal accomplishment. This scale has several versions, including the MBI-GS, which was the version developed in 1996 to cover all professional categories. However, this scale had a number of flaws, such as the possibility of bias in responses and the fact that the exhaustion dimension only measures affective aspects, ignoring physical and cognitive aspects of work.

The OLBI was created to overcome some of the psychometric limitations of the previous scale, which is based on the dimensions of exhaustion and disconnection from work, each with 8 (eight) questions. The scale uses a Likert-type structure for responses, ranging from 1 (one) to 4 (four), with 1 (one) being strongly disagree and 4 (four) being strongly agree.

The exhaustion dimension is defined as a consequence of intense affective and physical pressure, i.e. as a long-term consequence of certain unfavorable work demands. The disconnection from work dimension refers to distancing oneself from the object and content of the work, particularly with regard to identification with the work and the desire to remain in the same profession.

Despite the efforts made to expand studies on Burnout around the world, only in recent years has it begun to be studied with greater emphasis in Brazil. As a result, there was a need to adapt the scale to the working conditions and reality of our country and, therefore, studies aimed at validating the OLBI scale in Brazil.

As a result, it was necessary to exclude three variables (questions) that showed measurement mismatches. After the validation process, the scale was structured into six variables for checking the exhaustion factor (EE) and seven variables for the disconnection from work factor (DT). With thirteen questions (see table below), the scale showed an improvement on the model proposed by OLBI.

Thus, the validation of the OLBI scale in Brazil to measure Burnout provides the opportunity to develop new studies in the area of workers' health and the possibility of reducing the consequences of this syndrome, which is responsible for problems of various kinds, with impacts inside and outside organizations (SCHUSTER; DIAS, 2018).

Variables	Factor
I often do new and interesting things at work	DTI
More and more often I speak negatively about my work	DT2
Lately, I've been doing my work almost mechanically	DT3
I consider my work a positive challenge	DT4
Over time, I've become disinterested in my work	DT5
I feel more and more committed to my work	DT7
I often feel fed up with my tasks	DT8
Some days I feel tired before I even get to work	EEI
After work, I need more time to feel better than I used to	EE2
I can withstand the pressures of my job very well	EE3
During my work, I feel emotionally drained	EE4
After work, I have energy for my leisure activities	EE5
After work, I feel tired and low on energy	EE7

Prevention

Preventing Burnout Syndrome involves changing the organizational mentality at work. The development, promotion and implementation of health policies in the workplace is a matter of responsibility for workers' health.

Nowadays, the importance of occupational health services in the quest to expand research into occupational accidents and illnesses and the activities carried out to prevent and promote the health of workers in the labor market is clear. Their physical and mental health is fundamental in determining the progress of society (MUROFUSE; ABRANCHES; NAPOLEAO, 2005).

It is therefore necessary to think about workers' health and propose changes in the formulation of policies that protect and promote their health, which is fundamental to society and, of course, to collective health.

According to Franga and Rodrigues (1997, apud BARBOSA; OLIVEIRA; RIBEIRO, 2010), one of the ways to prevent the occurrence of Burnout Syndrome is to adopt measures to reduce predisposing factors such as psychological pressures; to try to maintain a variety in the routine of the work environment, avoiding monotony; to sustain social and organizational working conditions that are consistent with the work; and to avoid excessive overtime and long working hours.

It is recommended that institutions invest in the professional and personal development of workers and improve social support for them, providing spaces for workers to discuss the effects of organizational stress and come up with alternatives to mitigate the effects (NEVES; OLIVEIRA; ALVES, 2014).

Studies that encourage self-knowledge, structuring free time with pleasurable and attractive activities, periodic assessment of individual quality of life, assessment of individual limits of tolerance and demand, seeking less conflictive coexistence with peers and groups, reviewing and re-dimensioning forms of work organization, improving knowledge of their medical and social problems and concomitant economic, social and health planning are some of the measures that help prevent this syndrome (MOURAO et al., 2017). Annual monitoring of these workers is suggested, through interventions so that pathologies do not arise in the health of these employees caused by Burnout syndrome, as well as the improvement of continuing education, through educational lectures, based on risk analysis and the potential for these problems to appear (SIMOES; BIANCHI, 2016).

In addition, it is important to set up psychological care services and create multidisciplinary teams that are able to deal with work-related illnesses, with awareness of the vulnerabilities and limitations of each professional (LUZ et al., 2017).

It is also considered a strategy for institutions to adopt practices that allow professionals to participate effectively in decisions related to the organization's work process and the context of each patient's treatment, valuing their knowledge and the importance of their role as a member of a multidisciplinary team.

It is also very important to reconcile professional activities with leisure, physical activity and personal and social life, establishing links to avoid stress, rest and replenish energy.

For this to happen, it is essential that the category is valued, with compatible pay and adequate conditions for nursing work, focused on integrated care, articulated between the care and surveillance sectors.

The organizational culture must take a coherent and responsible stance, favoring the execution of preventive activities and contributing to the promotion of workers' health (BARBOSA; OLIVEIRA; RIBEIRO, 2010). Given this need for prevention, it is important to investigate the prevalence of Burnout in different professional categories and with different characteristics, pointing out possible proposals and more consistent interventions in order to minimize the onset of this disorder (SILVA; NORA; OLIVEIRA, 2017). From this, it is possible to alert society and managers to its relevance and the importance of implementing means to improve working conditions.

In this way, environments are created that foster the appreciation and recognition of these professionals. Some aspects need to be considered and analyzed, such as: possible reductions in working hours, more breaks and adequate space for rest, restructuring of the health team, especially with regard to a sufficient number of professionals, in order to reduce the wear and tear associated with emotional work and consequent turnover and burnout among nursing professionals.

It should be noted that working conditions are essential for satisfaction and health in the workplace and are fundamental to the quality of care.

Therefore, a two-pronged strategy is needed in order to retain nurses within the profession: a decrease in the demand for work, coupled with an increase in the use of available resources.

These are just some of the interventions that can be adopted by health institutions, which will in turn depend on the particular needs of each work environment and each worker.

3 MATERIAL AND METHODS

This study is a literature review with a qualitative, descriptive methodological approach. The research consists of analyzing previous relevant studies and discussing the theoretical framework of conceptual aspects relevant to the issue. To this end, we consulted articles and scientific journals, monographs, theses and dissertations in the Bireme and Medline databases, using the keywords burnout, nursing services and occupational health as descriptors. A total of 450 articles were made available and 23 of these were used. The inclusion criteria were articles related to the topic in the nursing category and the exclusion criteria were articles that dealt with other professional categories. In this way, description, comparison, analysis and synthesis were incorporated as elaboration techniques to construct the proposed objective. The research was carried out from March to July 2010 and was completed in 2018.

4. FINAL CONSIDERATIONS

The technological changes introduced by the work production process, easy access to information, the globalization of the economy and unemployment are very present in reality and have had significant impacts on workers' health with a view to increasing productivity, specifically for nursing professionals.

Acting, competent and effective professionals are intensely sought after as a matter of survival in the competitive market. This professional profile, which is considered suitable for the highly demanding organizational system, has also led to greater internal and external demands in order to achieve the ideal that is accepted and recognized as valid.

This scenario of change and uncertainty favors the emergence of anxiety, anguish, impotence and diminished self-esteem in the face of so many idealized attributions. Not being able to meet these demands can lead to psychosomatic illnesses due to the incompatibility of living up to the official standard, giving rise to psychic suffering.

In addition, it is clear that the nursing profession is permeated by constant challenges, which require the professional to have an immense adaptive capacity in the face of different situations and emergency conditions, a fact that can favor the development of illnesses and disorders such as Burnout Syndrome.

The increase in the number of cases of this syndrome, which is highly prevalent among nursing professionals, is worrying and is considered an international problem, corroborating the need for better knowledge and more in-depth research on the subject, as well as the interest of all professionals to understand this syndrome, which affects the nursing sector and is increasingly present in society.

Knowing that Burnout Syndrome is the result of a negative interaction in relation to working conditions and organization resulting from professional experience in a context of complex social relationships, involving the person's representation of themselves and others, and considering the individual and collective consequences derived from the illness, it is necessary to pay greater attention to these professionals.

Studying the syndrome has enabled us to understand and elucidate some of the most common occupational problems faced by nursing professionals, as well as allowing us to look for interventions for Burnout.

The consequences of burnout-turnover affect both professionals and organizations, leading to costs such as hiring staff, training, medical expenses and the loss of a qualified workforce. Thus, considering the combination of nursing demand and recurrent turnover behaviors, it is natural for nursing team managers to be increasingly concerned about the health of their team members and the quality of care provided to patients.

This involves greater support from their supervisors, with the development of policies that take into account the quality of life of these professionals. In addition, there is value in knowing and valuing the characteristics and stressors, manifestations and consequences of Burnout from the perspective of the nursing professionals themselves, as well as the strategies for preventing it.

These measures would help to draw up proposals for improvements to reduce the damage caused by this occupation and, consequently, to preserve health, as well as the possibility of better coping with the disease.

In this way, it can be seen that the increase in interest in Burnout coincides with concerns about quality of life and conceptual changes in health, contributing to the raising of critical questions about the subject and the expansion of scientific production and related research in this area, which are currently still scarce. Thus, developing an action plan for its prevention seems to be a challenge.

Most research of this type aims to carry out individual interventions, aimed at behavioral changes rather than changes at work, which is the origin of the syndrome.

If this is a worldwide trend, as research shows, Brazil needs to be prepared to face it, in order to preserve the well-being of the nursing staff, the comfort of patients and the proper functioning of healthcare institutions.

It is therefore suggested that future research study these variables in the Brazilian reality, in order to contribute to greater knowledge, prevention and treatment of the relationship between Burnout in nursing professionals in Brazil.

5 BIBLIOGRAPHICAL REFERENCES

ABRANCHES, S.S; MUROFUSE, N.T.; NAPOLEAO, A.A. Reflexoes Sobre Estresse e Burnout e a Relação com a Enfermagem. **Rev. Latino Enfermagem**, v. 13, n. 2, p. 255-261. Mar/Apr. 2005.

ARAUJO, M.B.J. et al. Burnout syndrome in residents of the Federal University of Uberlandia. **Rev. bras. educ. med.** [online], Rio de Janeiro, v. 31, n.2, p. 137-146. May/Aug. 2007.

AZEVEDO, B.D.S; NERY, A.A; CARDOSO, J.P. Estresse ocupacional e insatisfaçao com a qualidade de vida no trabalho da enfermagem. **Texto contexto - enferm**. Florianopolis, v.26, n.1,2017.[Online version]. ISSN 1980-265X. Disponlvel em:Http://dx.doi.org/10.1590/0104-07072017003940015. Accessed on: 09 Apr 2018.

BARBOSA, J.A.; OLIVEIRA, M.S.; RIBEIRO, C.C. **Burnout Syndrome and Nursing: Literature Review.** Course Conclusion Paper presented to Universidade Paulista. Santos, 2008. Available at:http://www.webartigos.com. Accessed: May 31, 2010.

BARRETO, A.S. et al. Burnout syndrome: Systematics of a problem. **Enfermagem Revista**, v. 16, n. 3, p. 276-296. 2012.

BENEVIDES- PEREIRA, A.M.T. **Burnout: when work threatens the well-being of the worker**. Sao Paulo: Casa do Psicologo. 2002.

BERESIN, R.; BEZERRA, R.P. **The Burnout Syndrome in Pre-Hospital Rescue Team Nurses**. Study carried out at the Faculty of Nursing of Hospital Israelita Albert Einstein - HIAE, Sao Paulo (SP), Brazil, 2009. Available at: http://apps.einstein.br/revista/arquivos/PDF/1186-Einstein%20v7n3p351-6 port.pdfAccessed: April 21, 2010.

BOFF, V.B et al. The Incidence of Burnout Syndrome in Nursing Professionals. Proceedings of **the 58th annual meeting of the SBPC**, Florianopolis/SC, July. 2006.

BRAZIL, Ministry of Health. **Work-related diseases: manual of procedures for health services**. Brasilia: Ministry of Health. 2001.

BUCASIO, E. et al. Burnout in the Psychiatric Clinic: a case report. **Rev. Psiquiatr. Rio Gd. Sul** , Porto Alegre, v. 28, n. 03, p. 352- 356, Sep/Dec. 2006.

FALGUERAS, M.V. et al. Burnout and teamwork in primary care professionals. **Atencion Primaria**, v. 47, n. 1, p. 25 31. 2015

FERNANDES, L.S. et al. Burnout Syndrome in Nursing Professionals of an Intensive Care Unit. **Rev Fund Care Online**, v. 9, n. 2, p. 551-557. apr/jun. 2017.

FRANCA, F.M. et al. Burnout and labor aspects in the nursing staff of two medium-sized hospitals. **Revista Latino-Americana de Enfermagem**, v. 20, n. 5, p. 961-970. 2012.

FRANCA, S,P.S. et al. Predictors of Burnout Syndrome in nurses of pre-hospital emergency services. **Acta Paul Enferm**, v. 25, n. 1, p. 68-73. 2012.

GREGORY, S.T.; MENSER, T. Burnout Among Primary Care Physicians: A Test of the Areas of Worklife Model. **Journal of Healthcare Management**, v. 60, n. 2, p. 133. 2015.

JESUS, C.P. et al. A new contribution to the classification of stressors affecting nursing professionals. **Rev. Latino-Am. Enfermagem,** v. 25. 2017. [Accessed: Feb 19, 2018]; Available at http://www.scielo.org/php/index.php.DOI: http://dx.doi.org/10.1590/1518-8345.1240.2895.

HALLAK, J.E.C.; TENG, C. T; TRIGO, T.R. Sindrome de Burnout ou Estafa Profissional e os Transtornos Psiquiatricos. **Rev. psiquiatr. Clin, Sao Paulo,** v.34, n. 5, p. 223-233. 2007.

HADDAD, M.C.L.; JODAS, D. A. Burnout Syndrome in Nursing Workers at a University Hospital Emergency Room. **Acta paul. enferm.**, Sao Paulo, v. 22, n. 2, p. 192-197. 2009.

IACOVIDES, A. et al. The Relationship Between Job Stress, Burnout and Clinical Depression. **J Affect Disord**, v. 75, n. 3, p. 209-221. 2003.

LIMA, A.S; FARAH, B.F; BUSTAMANTE-TEIXEIRA, M.T. Analysis of the prevalence of burnout syndrome in primary health care professionals. **Trab. Educ. Saude**, Rio de Janeiro, v. 16 n. 1, p. 283-304, jan./abr. 2018.

LUZ, L. M. et al. Burnout Syndrome in Mobile Emergency Care Service Professionals. **Rev Fund Care Online**, v. 9, n. 1, p. 238-246. jan/mar. 2017.

LUZ, L. M. et al. Review of The Failure of the Project of Being: Burnout, Existence and Paradoxes of Work. **Rev. de Psicologia**, Fortaleza, v.8 n. 2, p. 183-184, jul./dez. 2017.

MASLACH, C; SCHAUFELI, W. C; LEITER, M. P. Job burnout. **Annu Rev. Psychol.** p. 397-422. 2001.

MEDEIROS-COSTA, M.E. et al. Occupational Burnout Syndrome in the nursing context: an integrative literature review. **Rev Esc Enferm USP,** v. 51. 2017. DOI: http://dx.doi.org/10.1590/S1980-220X2016023403235.

MOURAO, A.L. et al. Burnout Syndrome in the Nursing Context. **Rev. Baiana de Saude Publica**, v.41, n.1, p.131-143. 2017.

MUROFUSE, N.T.; ABRANCHES, S.S.; NAPOLEAO, A.A. Reflexoes sobre estresse e Burnout e a relagao com a enfermagem. **Revista Latino-Americana de Enfermagem**, v. 13, n. 2, p. 255-261, 2005.

NEVES, V.F.; OLIVEIRA, A.F.; ALVES, P.C. Burnout syndrome: impact of job satisfaction and perception of organizational support. **Psico**, v. 45, n. 1, p. 45-54. 2014.

PADILLHA, K.G. et al. Nursing workload, stress/burnout, satisfaction and incidents in a trauma intensive care unit. **Texto Contexto Enferm**, v. 26, n. 3. 2017.

PORTELA, N.L.C. et al. Burnout syndrome in nursing professionals in urgent and emergency care services. **Rev. pesqui. cuid. fundam.(Online)**, v. 7, n. 3, p. 2749-2760, 2015.

RITTER, R.S.; STUMM, E.M.F.; KIRCHER, R.M. Análise de Burnout em Profissionais de uma Unidade de Emergencia de um Hospital Geral. **Rev. Eletr. Enf,** v. 11, n.02, p. 236-248. 2009.

SCHAUFELI, W.B.; LEITER, M.P.; MASLACH, C. Burnout: 35 years of research and practice. **Career development international**, v. 14, n. 3, p. 204-220, 2009.

SCHUSTER, M.S; DIAS, V.V. Oldenburg Burnout Inventory - validation of a new way to measure Burnout in Brazil. **Ciencia & Saude Coletiva**, v. 23, n.2, p. 553-562. 2018. DOI: 10.1590/1413-81232018232.27952015.

SILVA, A.A; NORA, M; OLIVEIRA, M.Z. The predictive role of burnout syndrome for turnover in nursing professionals. **Avances en Psicologia Latinoamericana**, Bogota (Colombia), v, 35, n. 3, p. 433-445. 2017. ISSNe2145-4515.

SIMOES, J.; BIANCHI, L. R. O. Prevalence of *Burnout* Syndrome and Sleep Quality in Nursing Technician Workers. **Rev. Saude e Pesquisa,** Maringa (PR), v. 9, n. 3, p. 473-481, Sep./Dec. 2016.

TAMAYO, M.R. Burnout: Implications of Organizational Sources of Individual-Work Maladjustment in Nursing Professionals. **Psychol. Reflex. Crit.,** Porto Alegre, v. 22, n. 03, p. 474-482. 2009.

WORM, F. A. et al. Risk of Illness among Nursing Professionals Working in Mobile Emergency Care. **Rev. Cuid.,** v. 7, n. 2, p.1288-96. 2016.

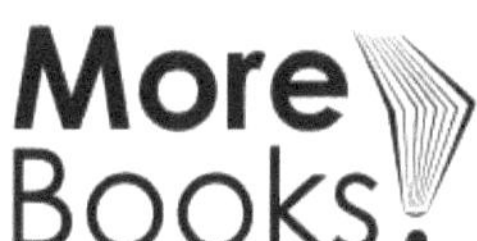

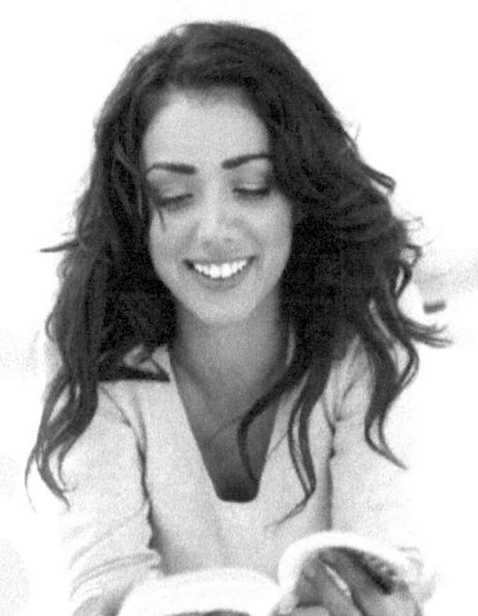

I want morebooks!

Buy your books fast and straightforward online - at one of world's fastest growing online book stores! Environmentally sound due to Print-on-Demand technologies.

Buy your books online at
www.morebooks.shop

Kaufen Sie Ihre Bücher schnell und unkompliziert online – auf einer der am schnellsten wachsenden Buchhandelsplattformen weltweit! Dank Print-On-Demand umwelt- und ressourcenschonend produziert.

Bücher schneller online kaufen
www.morebooks.shop

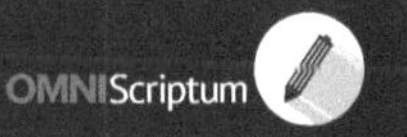